About the author

Lara Curran, the author with a deep understanding of the unique needs and consideration of age group, is specifically tailored for seniors over 60. I've carefully curated a collection of gentle and safe yoga routines that can be practiced comfortably from a chair or mat. My aim is to help older individuals enhance their physical and mental well-being through these age-appropriate exercises. The book is filled with heartfelt endeavors to promote flexibility, strength, and a sense of calm for seniors, empowering them to embrace a healthier and more active lifestyle.

Table of contents

Introduction

Welcome to the world of chair yoga, a gentle and effective practice designed especially for seniors aged 60 and above. As we journey through life, our bodies change, and so do our physical needs. Chair yoga offers a refreshing approach to physical and mental well-being, customized to fit the unique talents and requirements of elderly adults. Through a sequence of conscious movements, mild stretches, and breath-centered exercises, chair yoga helps seniors develop flexibility, balance, and relaxation while seated comfortably. Whether you're new to yoga or searching for a safe and accessible way to stay active, this book will encourage you to go on a journey of self-care and vitality, proving that age is no barrier to achieving a healthy mind and body.

Chapter 1

Definition and benefits of chair yoga

Chair yoga is a modified style of yoga that is designed to be practiced while sitting on a chair or utilizing a chair for support. It adjusts classic yoga postures and practices to assist people with restricted mobility, physical disabilities, or those who find it tough to practice yoga on the floor. Chair yoga offers a gentle and accessible approach to enjoying the benefits of yoga, making it particularly well-suited for seniors over the age of 60.

Benefits of Chair Yoga:

Improved Flexibility: Chair yoga contains a range of moderate stretches and motions that help to enhance flexibility in the muscles and joints. Over time, persistent practice can expand the range of motion and make daily activities more pleasant.

Enhanced Balance: Chair yoga poses often involve stability exercises that promote balance and coordination. Strengthening the muscles essential for balance helps lower the chance of falls, a significant concern among seniors.

Reduced Joint Strain: Chair yoga is meant to limit stress on the joints, making it perfect for seniors who might have joint difficulties or arthritis. The supporting quality of the chair allows people to engage in yoga positions without discomfort.

Stress Reduction: The breath-focused approach of chair yoga improves relaxation and relieves stress. Mindful breathing and relaxation techniques practiced during chair yoga sessions can have a calming effect on the neurological system, aiding in stress management.

Enhanced Circulation: The gentle motions and stretches in chair yoga encourage blood circulation throughout the body. This can help with blood flow to muscles and extremities, improving overall cardiovascular health.

Mind-Body Connection: Chair yoga stresses the connection between the body, breath, and mind. Seniors can experience a sense of mindfulness and presence during meditation, encouraging mental clarity and reducing anxiety.

Accessible Fitness: Chair yoga gives a fitness option for the elderly who may have problems with traditional exercise routines. It provides an opportunity to engage in physical activity without the need to get down on the floor or perform severe movements.

Community and Social Interaction: Group chair yoga courses give seniors a social outlet where they can engage with others who have similar goals. This sense of community can contribute to general well-being.

Suitability for Seniors Over 60:

Chair yoga is particularly well-suited for seniors over the age of 60 due to its gentle nature and adjustability. As individuals age, they may suffer changes in mobility, balance, and joint health. Chair yoga addresses these concerns by offering support and adjustments for diverse physical capacities. It avoids the possible difficulty of getting up and down from the floor, making it more accessible for older folks.

Furthermore, chair yoga takes into account typical health concerns that seniors could suffer from, such as arthritis, osteoporosis, and limited mobility. Poses can be changed to fit these limitations and provide a safe and productive practice. Seniors can experience the advantages of yoga without extra strain or the risk of harm.

Overall, chair yoga is an inclusive and versatile practice that encourages seniors to maintain and increase their well-being, even as they develop the natural changes that come with aging.

Chapter 2

Chair yoga techniques to improve flexibility

1. Seated Forward Fold:

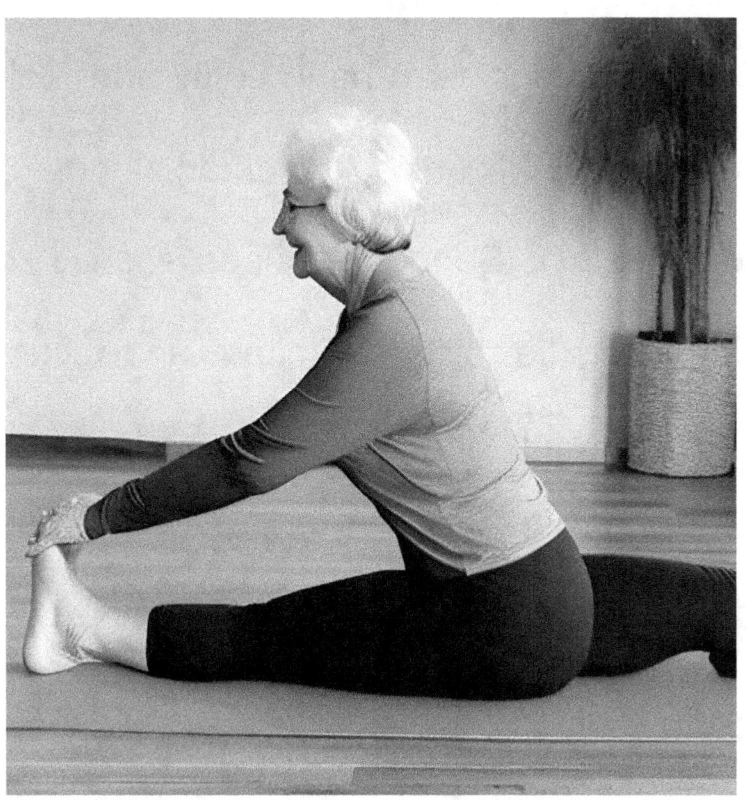

Sit on the edge of the chair with your feet flat on the floor.Inhale, stretch your spine, and exhale as you fold forward from your hips, reaching your hands towards the floor. Let your head hang softly and feel the stretch in your back and hamstrings. Modification: Bend the knees slightly if hamstring flexibility is limited, and focus on the stretch along the spine.

2. Seated Spinal Twist:

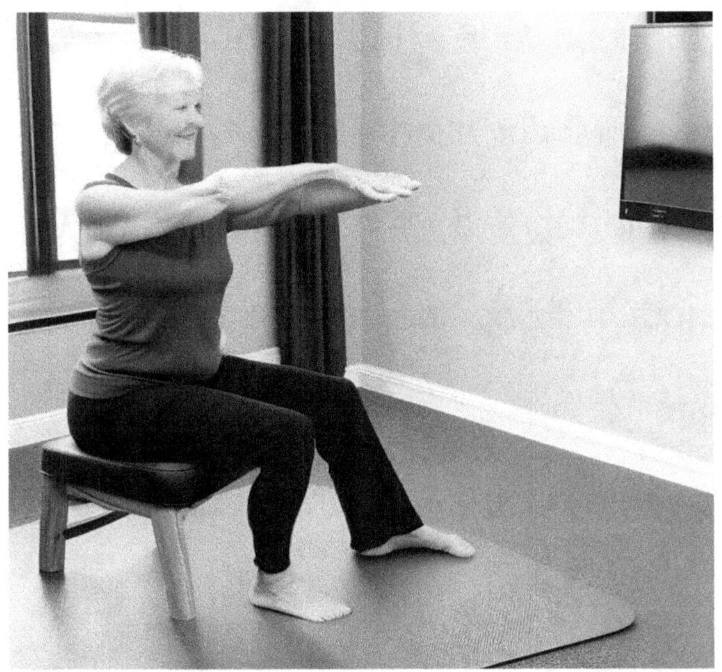

Sit sideways on the chair, grasping the backrest for support. Inhale, stretch your spine, and exhale as you gently twist your torso to one side, using your hand on the chair for leverage. Feel the stretch throughout your spine and through your core. Modification: If twisting is uncomfortable, try a modest seated twist without utilizing the arm to deepen the twist.

3. Seated Wide-Legged Stretch:

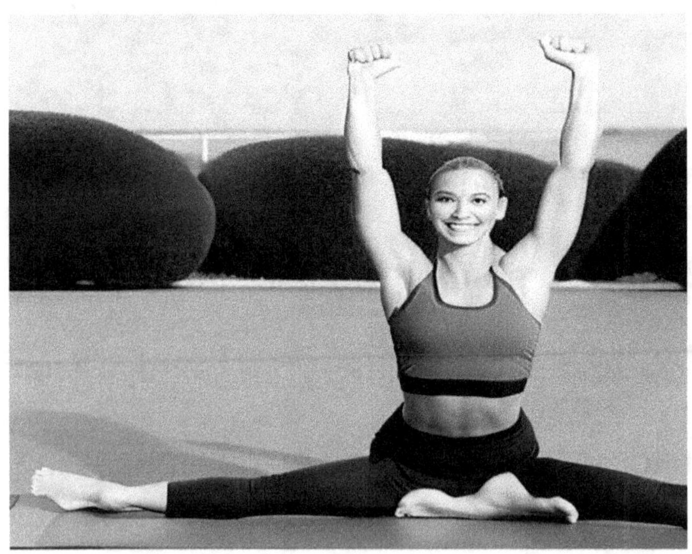

Sit on the chair with your legs wide apart. Inhale and stretch your spine, then exhale and gradually tilt forward from your hips, keeping your back straight. Reach your hands towards the floor or your shins, feeling the stretch in your inner thighs and hamstrings.

Modification: Adjust the leg posture to allow comfort and emphasize the stretch around the inner thighs.

4. Seated Pigeon Pose:

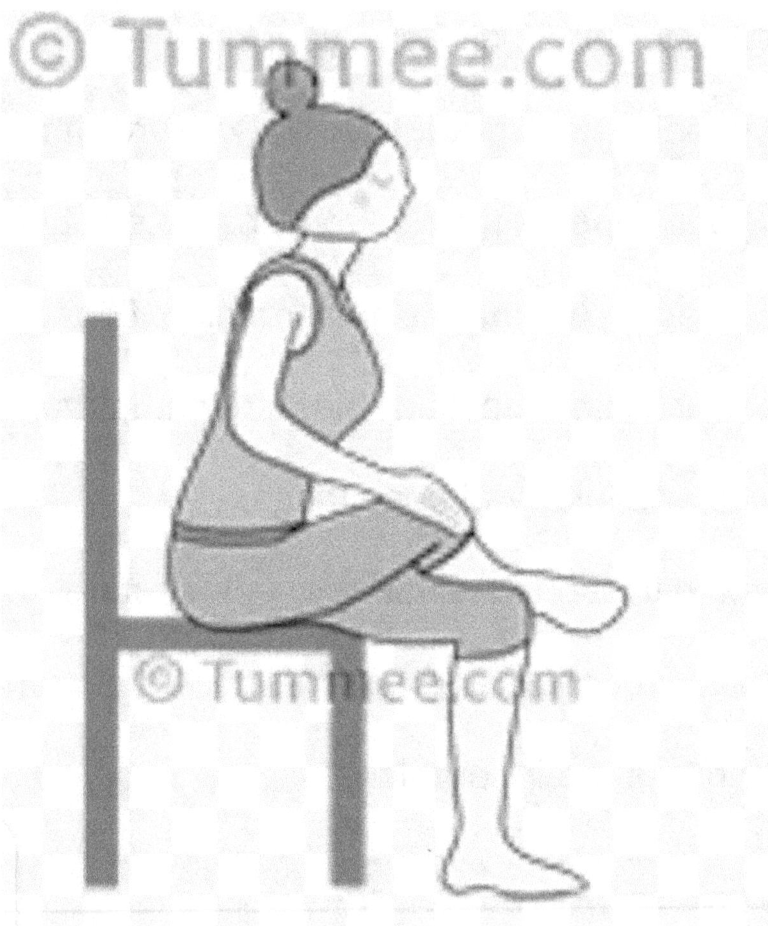

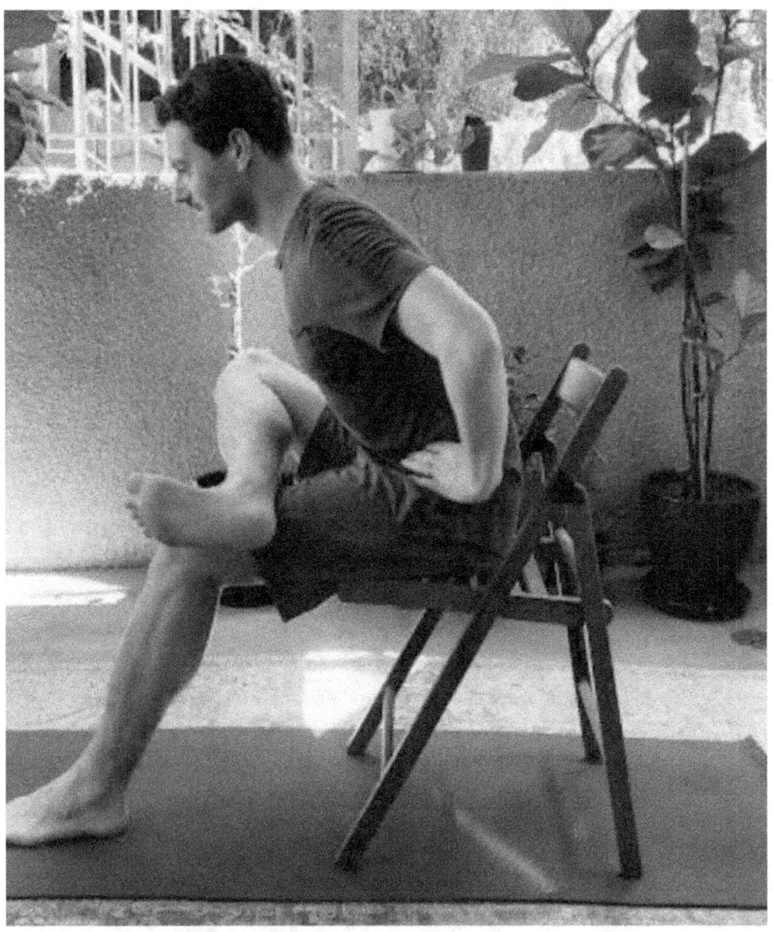

Sit on the edge of the chair with one ankle resting on the opposite knee.Press gently on the raised knee to feel a stretch in the hip of the raised leg.Switch sides to stretch both hips.Modification: If hip mobility is limited, place the ankle on the thigh or shin rather than the knee.

5. Seated Cat-Cow Stretch

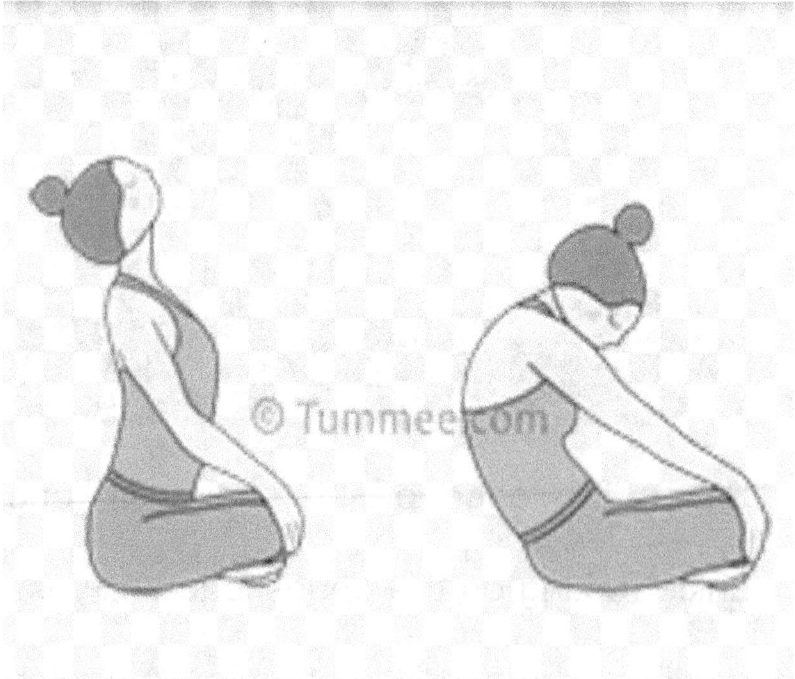

Sit erect with hands on your knees. Inhale, arch your back (cow), elevate your chest, and look up.Exhale and circle your back (cat), tucking your chin to your chest. Move through these motions with your breath, focusing on spinal flexibility.

Modification: Perform smaller spinal movements if rounding the back is problematic, focusing on the soft arch.

6. Seated Shoulder Opener:

Sit comfortably and interlace your fingers behind your back. Gently lift your arms away from your body, experiencing a stretch in your chest and shoulders. This stretch helps increase upper-body flexibility.

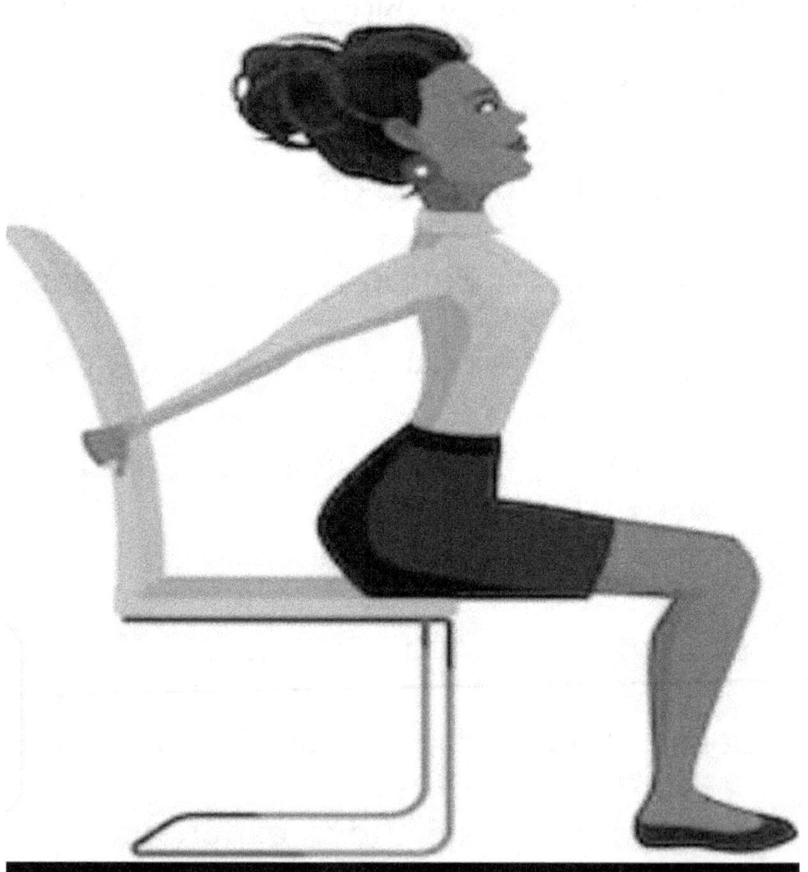

Modification: If reaching the arm is difficult, use a towel or strap to bridge the gap between the hands. Remember, flexibility increases gradually over time. Encourage seniors to breathe deeply and relax into each stretch, avoiding any pain. Always prioritize comfort and safety in their practice, and encourage them to utilize cushions or props for support if needed. If they have any medical issues, recommend visiting a healthcare expert before starting a new fitness plan.

Chapter 3

Exercises for balance enhancement

1. Seated leg lifts:

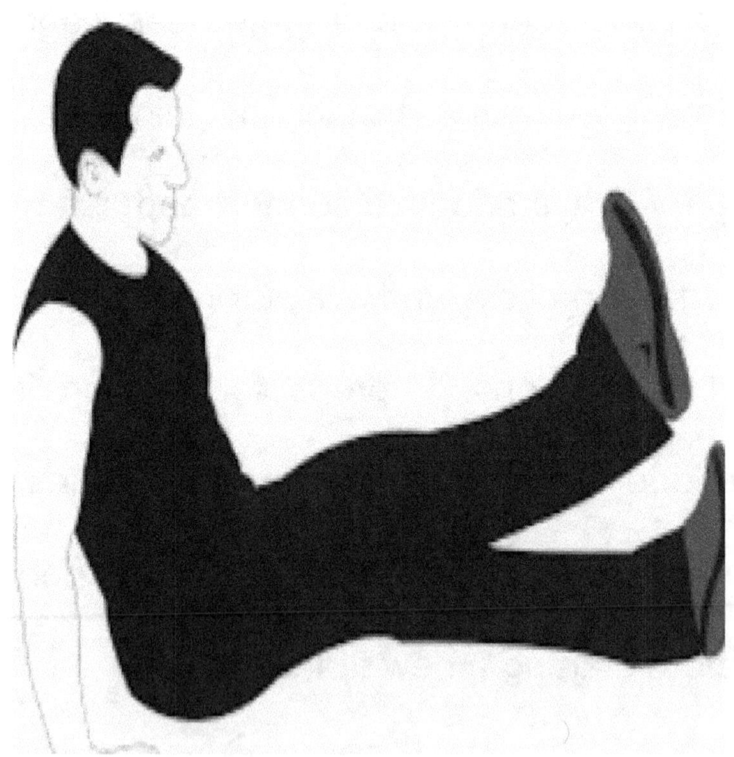

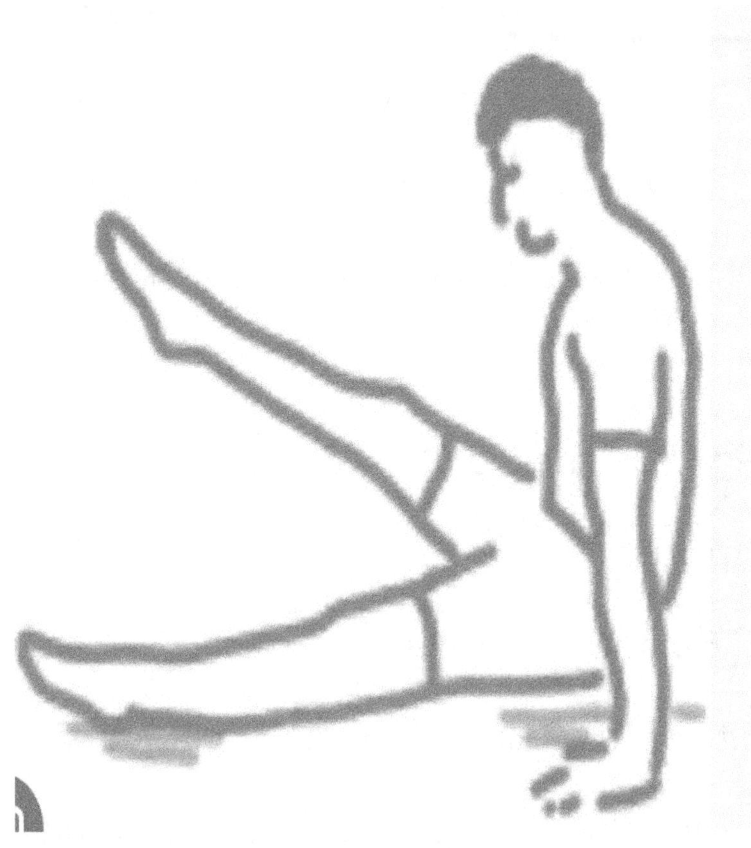

Sit comfortably with your feet level on the

floor and your hands resting on your

thighs. Lift one leg straight out in front of

you, holding it for a few breaths. Lower the leg and repeat with the opposite leg. This workout challenges your equilibrium while seated.Modification: Hold onto the chair or wall for support while lifting the leg, or lift the leg only a few inches off the ground.

2. Seated Tree Pose:

Sit with a straight spine and your feet flat on the floor. Lift one foot off the ground and place the sole against the inner thigh of the opposite leg. Find your balance and hold for a few breaths before transferring to the other leg.

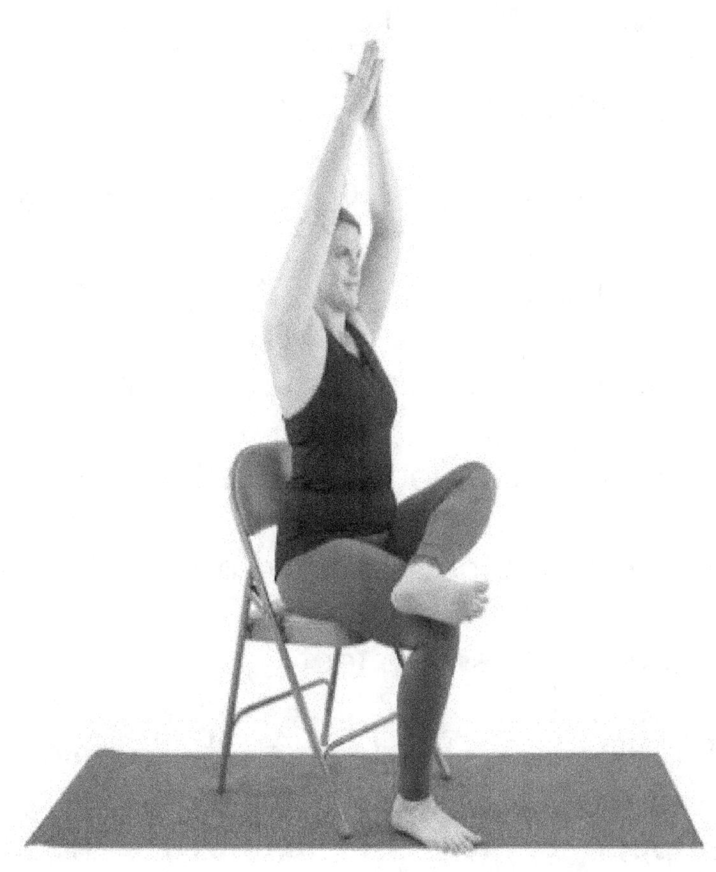

Modification: Keep the foot resting against the lower leg rather than pressing it high on the thigh.

3. Seated Tightrope Walk:

Sit with your feet flat on the floor and your hands on your thighs. Imagine walking on a tightrope. Lift one foot slightly off the floor and position it in front of the other foot. Balance on one foot for a time, then switch feet.

Modification: Hold onto the chair for support or perform the move with both feet touching the ground.

4. Seated Warrior III Variation:

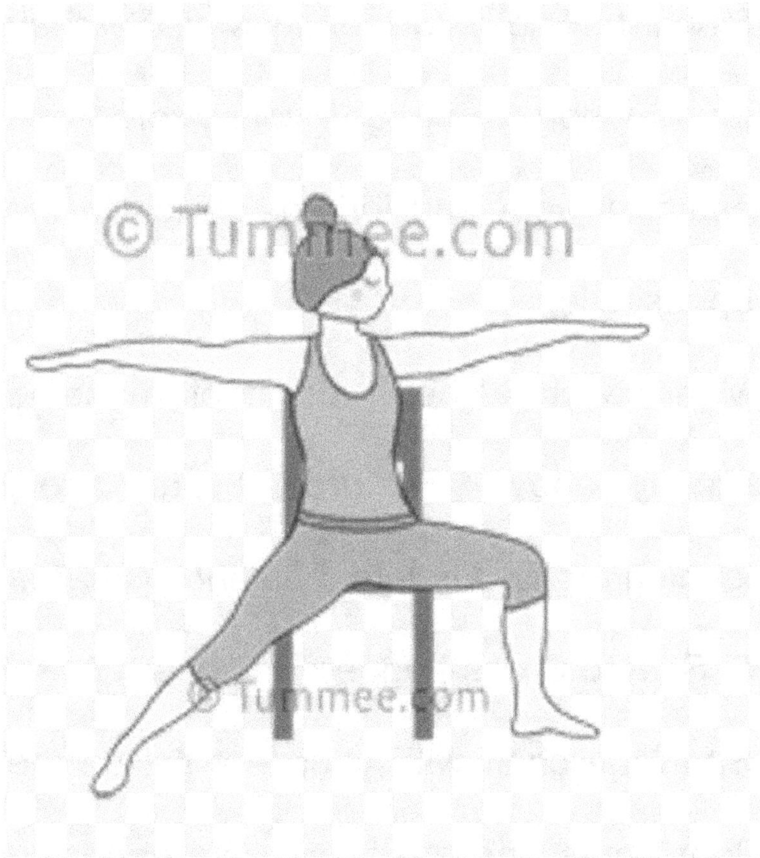

Sit at the edge of the chair with your spine straight. Extend one leg straight out in front of you while leaning slightly forward. Hold onto the sides of the chair for support. Engage your core and establish your equilibrium. Switch to the opposite leg.

Modification: Keep the foot hanging slightly above the ground and avoid leaning too far forward if balance is hard.

5. Seated Cross-Legged Balance:

Sit in the chair with your feet flat on the floor.Cross one ankle over the opposing knee.Gently press down on the lifted knee to work your hip muscles and challenge your balance.Switch to the opposite leg.Modification: Use the hand on the chair for support while balancing on one leg.

6. Seated heel lifts:

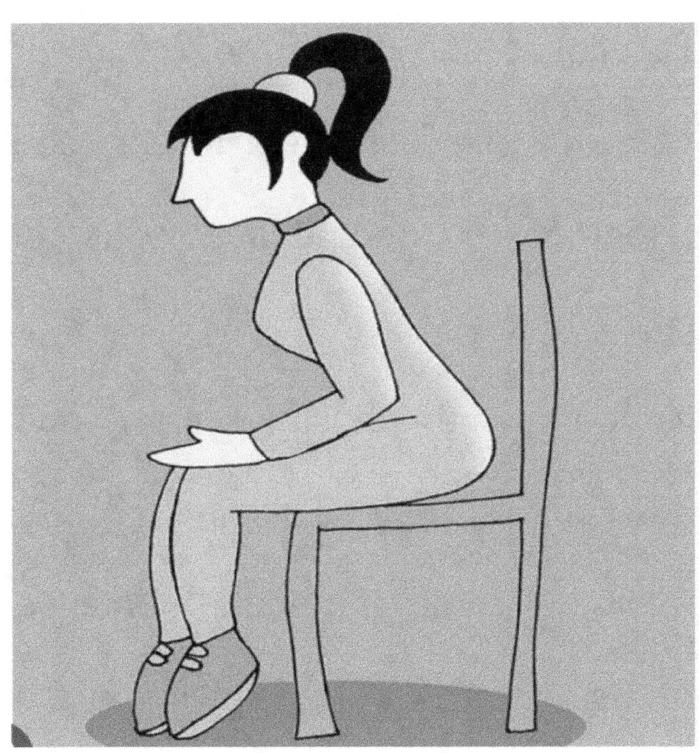

Sit with your feet flat on the floor and your hands on your thighs. Lift your heels off the ground, balancing on the balls of your feet. Hold for a second, then lower your heels back down.

Modification: Hold onto the chair for support while executing heel lifts, or keep both feet on the ground and focus on elevating the toes.

Remember to emphasize safety and provide support, such as holding onto the back of the chair, if needed. Balance exercises should be practiced in a regulated manner to prevent falls or discomfort. If elders have any medical concerns that influence their balance, encourage them to visit a healthcare expert before undertaking new exercises.

Chapter 4

chair yoga exercises to reduce joint pain

1. Seated Ankle Circles:

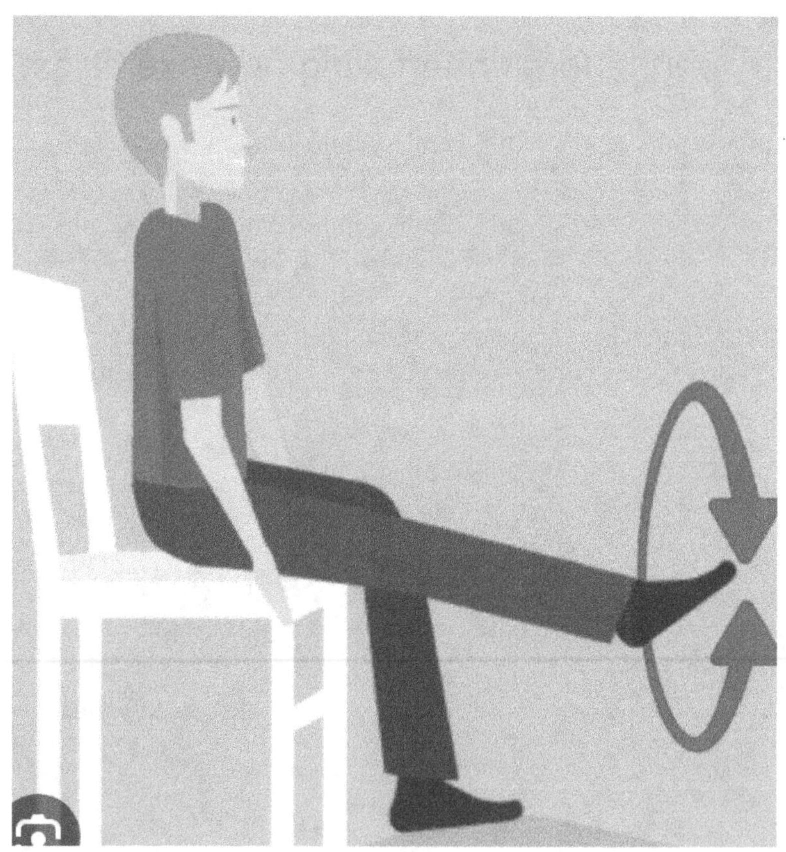

Sit comfortably with your feet level on the floor. Lift one foot off the ground and gently rotate your ankle in a circular motion. Perform several circles in each direction, then transfer to the other foot. Modification: Perform smaller circles and minimize the range of motion if ankle mobility is limited.

2. Seated Knee Hugs:

Sit with a straight spine and your heels flat on the floor. Hug one knee towards your torso, holding it gently.Release and transfer to the other knee. This exercise can help release tension in the hips and legs.

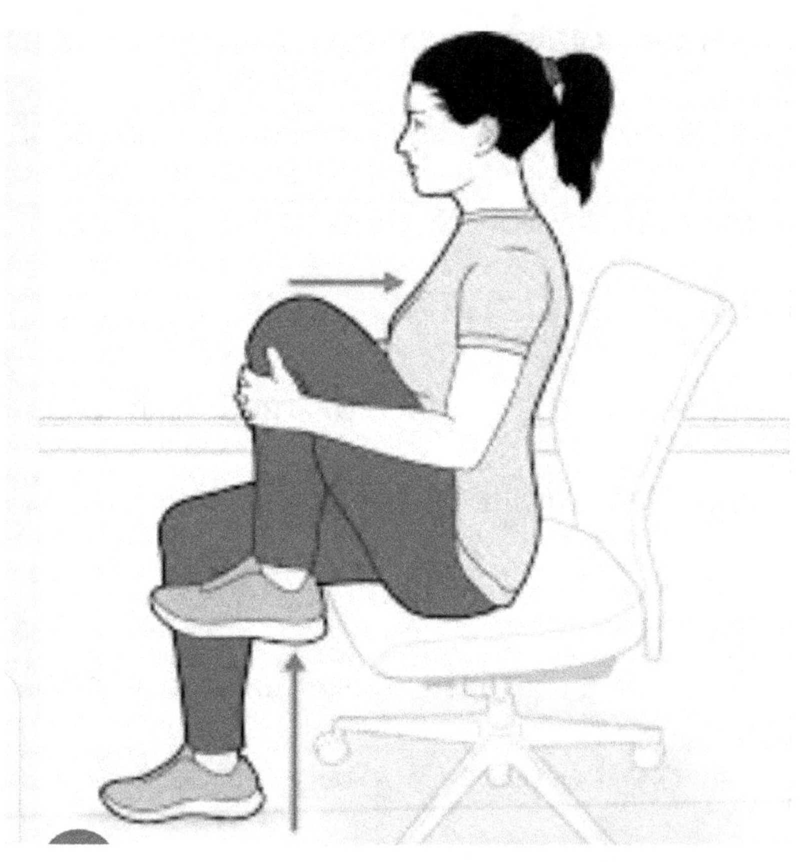

Modification: For those with limited hip flexibility, hold onto the back of the thigh rather than pulling the leg close.

3. Seated Shoulder Rolls:

Sit comfortably with your palms resting on your thighs.Inhale as you raise your shoulders up towards your ears.Exhale and rotate your shoulders back and down.Repeat this rolling motion several times to release tension in the shoulders.Modification: If raising the shoulders is uncomfortable, simply execute backward shoulder rolls while seated upright.

4. Seated Chest Opener:

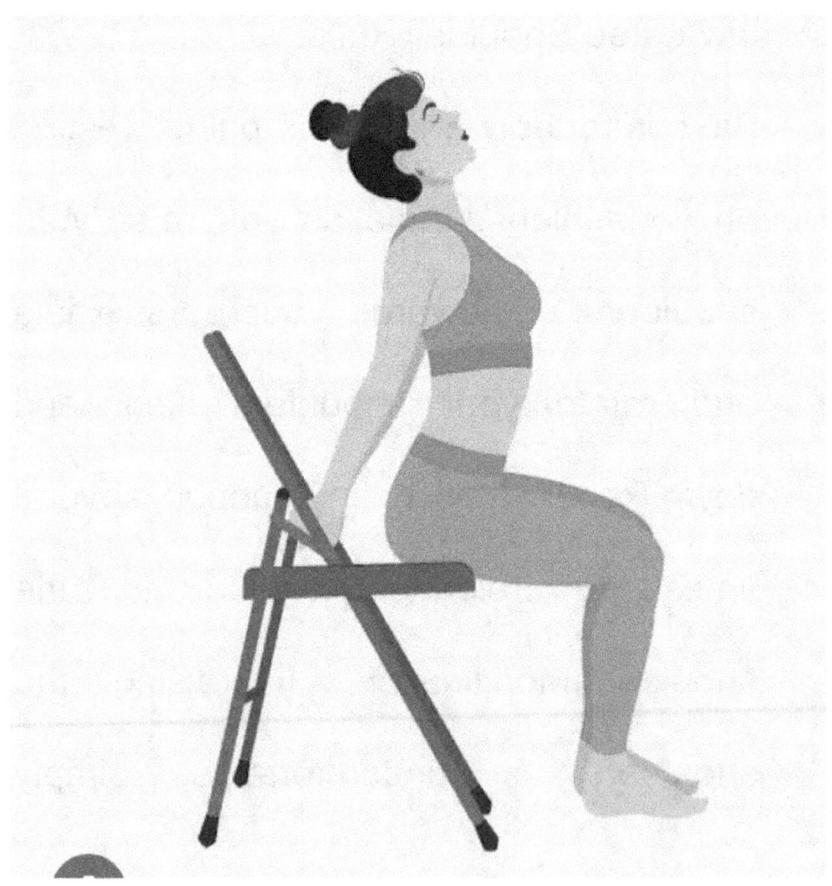

Sit at the edge of the chair with your hands linked behind your back. Gently lift your arms away from your body, opening your torso. Hold for a few breaths, then release.

Modification: If clasping hands is challenging, hold onto a belt or strap behind the back to accomplish the chest opening.

5. Seated Forward Fold Variation:

Sit on the chair with your feet level on the floor. Interlace your fingers behind your back and gently lift your arms as you fold forward. This provides a mild stretch to the shoulders and reduces strain on the lower back.

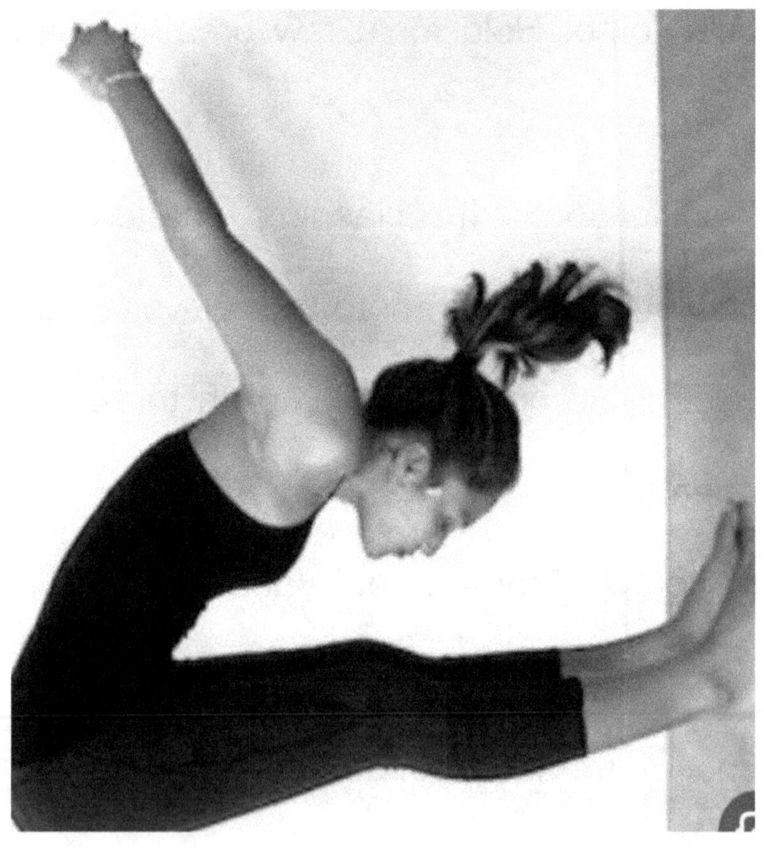

Modification: For those with back issues, merely fold forward gently without interlacing the fingers.

6. Seated Spinal Twist with Gentle Reach:

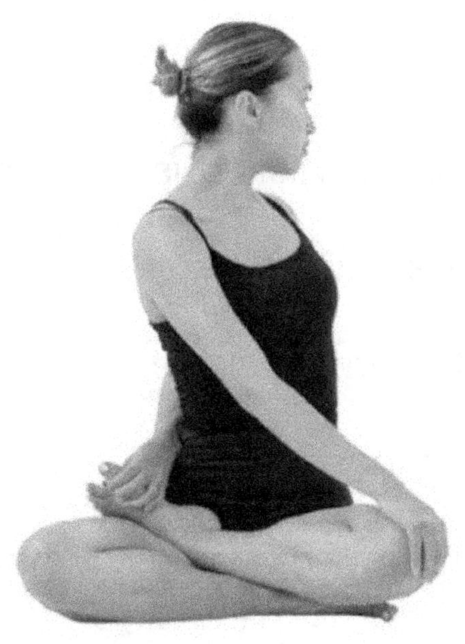

Sit sideways on the chair, gripping the backrest for support. Inhale and lengthen your spine, then exhale as you gently rotate your torso. Reach the opposite arm upwards to enhance the pirouette. This helps relieve tension in the spine and shoulders.

Modification: If twisting is uncomfortable, execute a seated side stretch by gently reaching the arm over the head.

Always remind seniors to move gently and avoid any movements that cause distress or pain. Chair yoga should be done mindfully and without strain. Encourage them to use cushions or objects for added support and to consult with a healthcare professional if they have any concerns or existing joint issues.

Chapter 5

Chair yoga exercises to reduce stress

1. Deep Breathing:

Sit comfortably in the chair with your spine erect. Close your eyes and take a few deep, deliberate breaths. Inhale thoroughly through your nose, expanding your abdomen. Exhale steadily through your mouth. Focus on your breath, letting go of any tension with each exhalation.

Modification: If deep breaths are challenging, promote slow, gentle breaths without focusing on deep inhalations.

2. Seated Forward Fold with Relaxation:

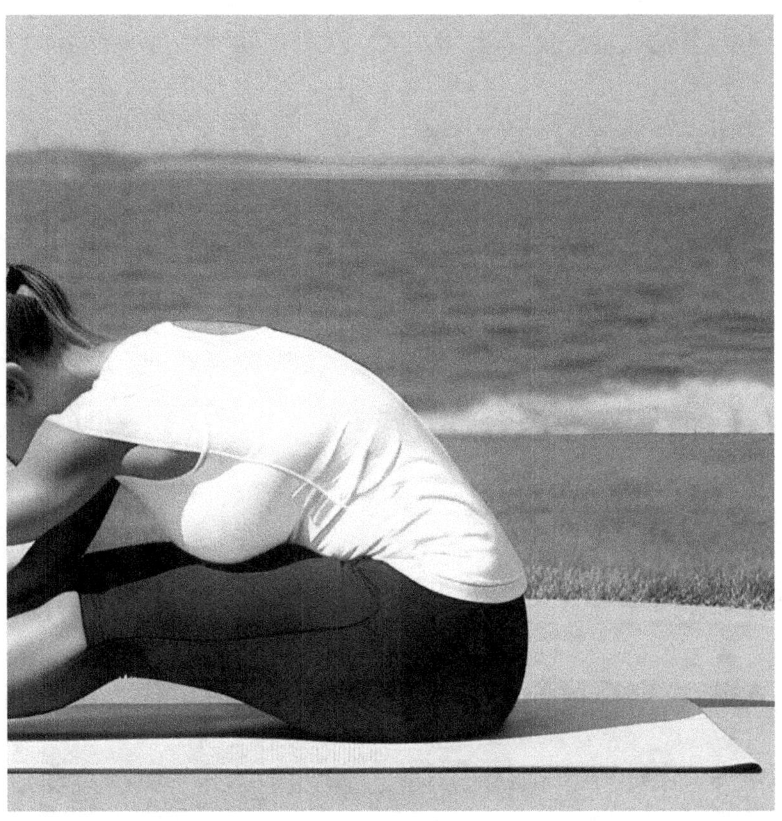

Sit on the edge of the chair with your feet level on the floor. Inhale and lengthen your spine, then exhale as you gently fold forward, allowing your arms to hang. Close your eyes and relax into the stretch for a few long breaths. Modification: For those with limited flexibility, merely lean forward slightly and focus on relaxation.

3. Seated Neck and Shoulder Release:

Sit comfortably and unwind your shoulders. Inhale as you elongate your spine, and as you exhale, gently tilt your head to the side, bringing your ear towards your shoulder.You can also use your hand to add a gentle stretch by applying slight pressure to the opposite side of your cranium.

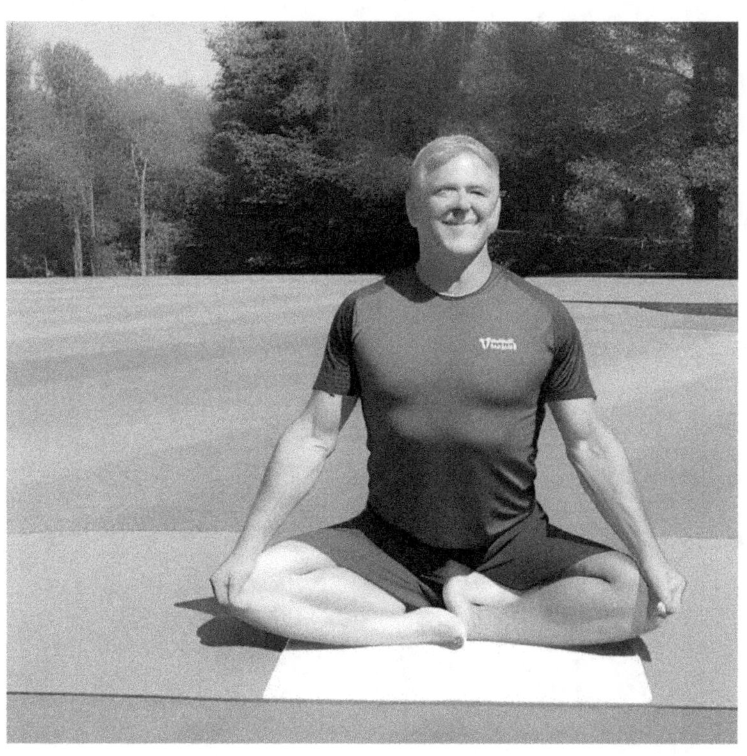

Modification: If neck mobility is limited, execute gentle neck tilts without pressing on the head.

4. Seated Sun Breath:

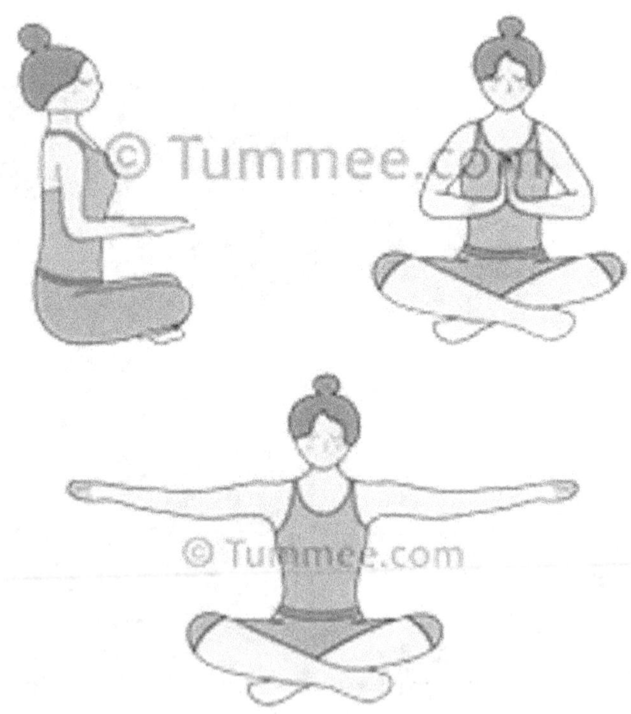

Sit with an erect spine and inhale as you sweep your arms overhead. Exhale and bring your palms down in front of your heart, simulating a "sunrise" motion. Inhale, reach your arms up again, and exhale to lower them back down. Coordinate each movement with your respiration.Modification: Keep the arm movements smaller and less exaggerated if elevating the arms is uncomfortable.

5. Guided Visualization:

Sit comfortably with your eyes closed. Imagine a serene and peaceful location, like a calm beach or a quiet forest. Visualize yourself there, focusing on the sights, sounds, and sensations. Let yourself relax and let go of tension.

Modification: Simplify the visualization by focusing on one relaxing image or sensation.

6. Relaxing Hand and Finger Stretches:

Extend your arms directly in front of you. Gently spread your fingers apart, then compress them into a fist. Open and close your fingers several times, then gently rotate your wrists in both directions.

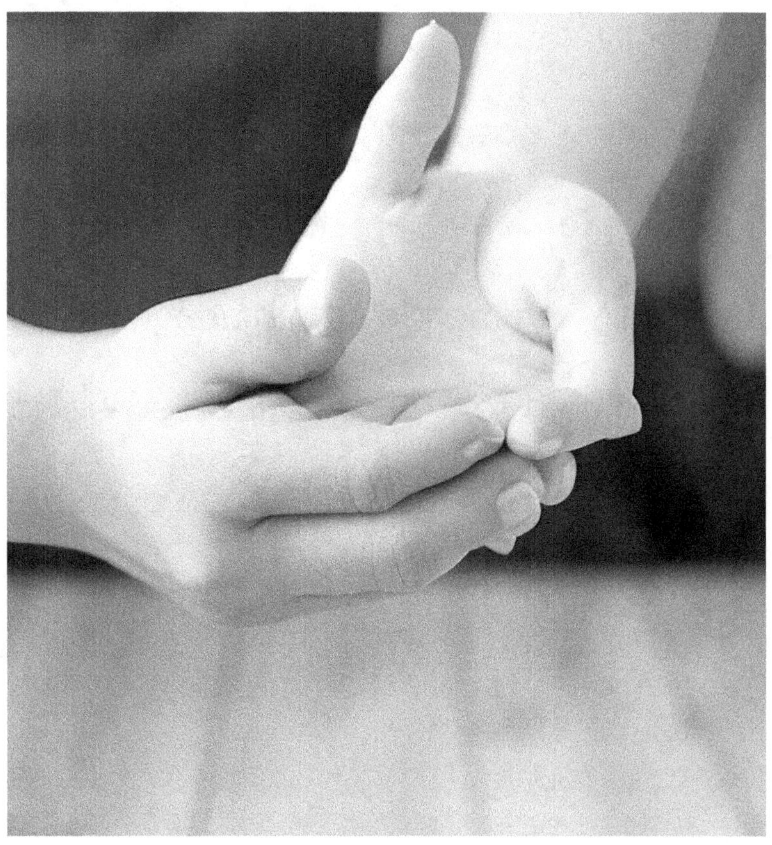

Modification: Perform gentle hand movements without exerting yourself if joint mobility is limited.

Encourage seniors to move slowly and mindfully, focusing on their respiration and letting go of any stress or tension. These exercises can be integrated into their daily regimen to help manage stress and promote relaxation. If they're new to chair yoga or have any concerns, suggest they consult with a healthcare professional before commencing a new exercise routine.

Chapter 6

Chair yoga exercises to enhance circulation

1. Seated Marching:

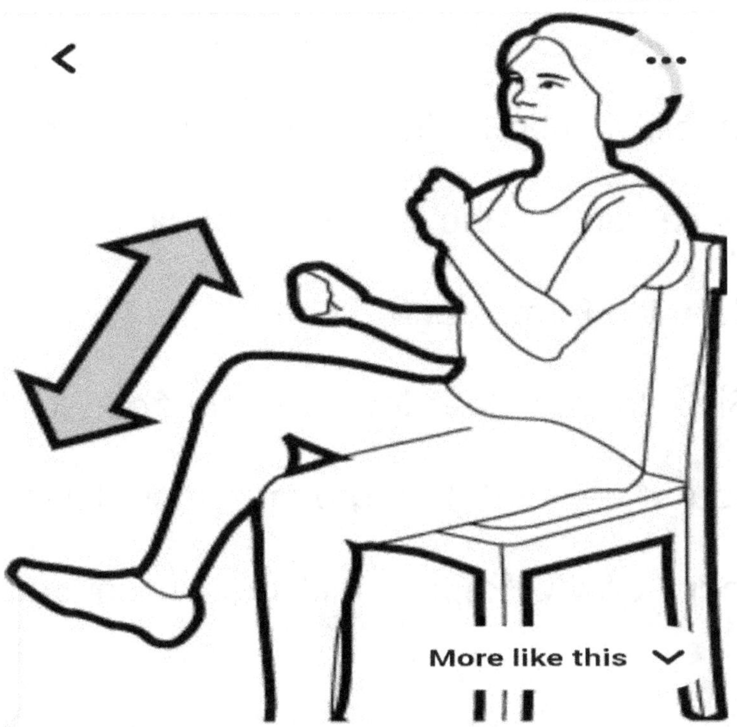

Sit at the edge of the chair with your feet level on the floor. Lift one knee up towards your torso and then lower it down. Alternate legs in a marching motion, engaging your core.

Modification: For those with limited mobility, merely lift the heels alternately while keeping the feet on the floor.

2. Ankle Pumps and Circle:

Sit with your feet level on the floor. Lift your heels off the ground, then lower them down. Repeat this motion several times. Next, rotate your ankles in circles, both clockwise and counterclockwise.

Modification: If ankle flexibility is limited, concentrate on ankle pumps (lifting and lowering) without performing circles.

3. Seated Forward Lean and Lift:

Sit with your feet level on the floor. Inhale and lengthen your spine, then exhale as you lean slightly forward from your pelvis. Inhale to elevate your chest and return to an upright position. This movement encourages blood flow to your extremities.

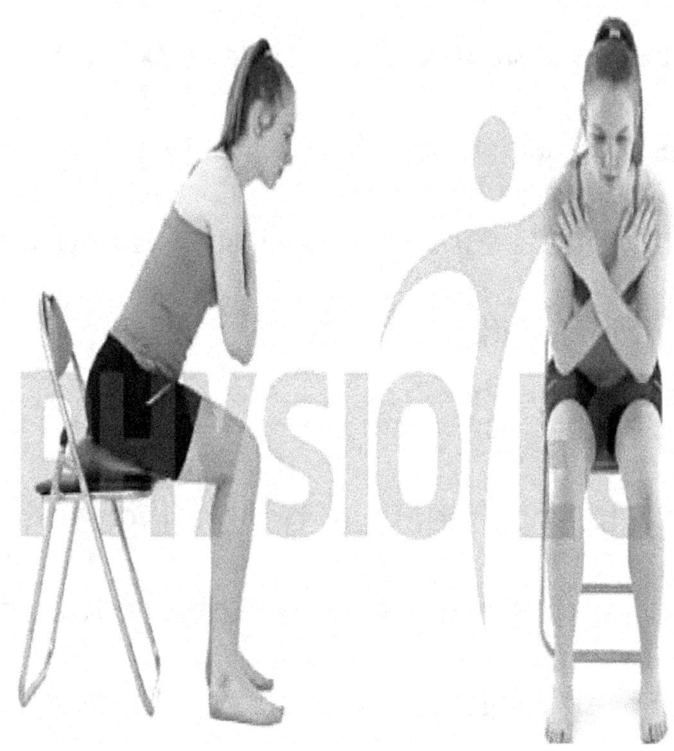

Modification: For those with balance concerns, merely sit upright and lift the feet off the ground one at a time.

4. Seated Arm Swings:

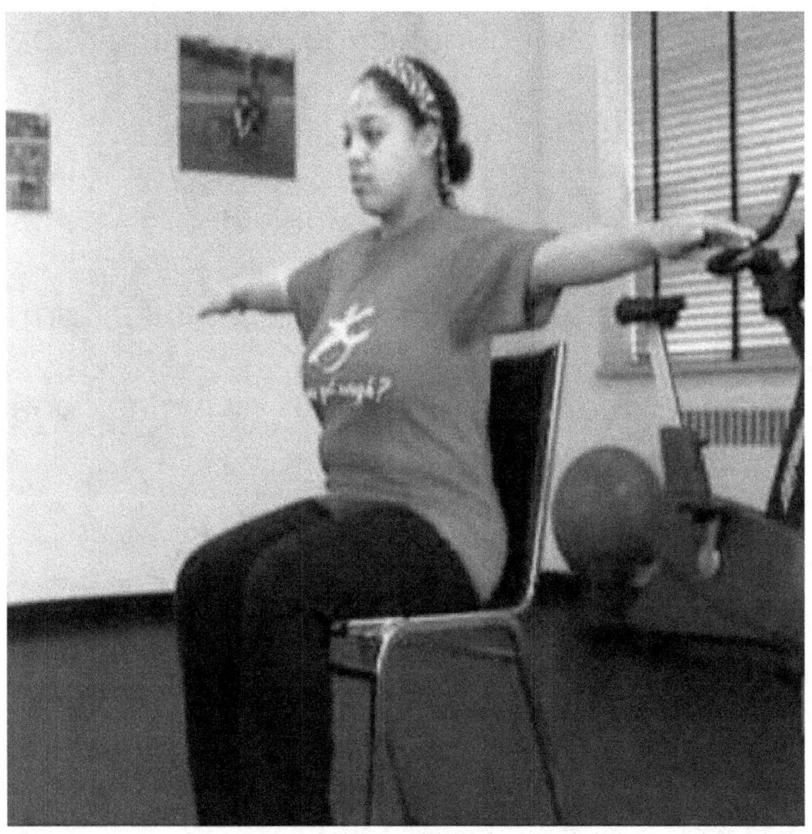

Sit comfortably and extend your arms out

to the sides. Swing your arms forward

and then back, as if you were swimming. This movement helps increase circulation in your upper body.

Modification: For individuals with shoulder issues, execute smaller arm movements or alternate swinging one arm at a time.

5. Seated Spinal Twist with Arm Circles: Sit comfortably and hold onto the sides of the chair for support. Inhale, lengthen your spine, and exhale as you gently rotate your torso. Extend your arms out to the sides and make small circles with

your arms in both directions. Repeat the

spiral and arm circles on the other side.

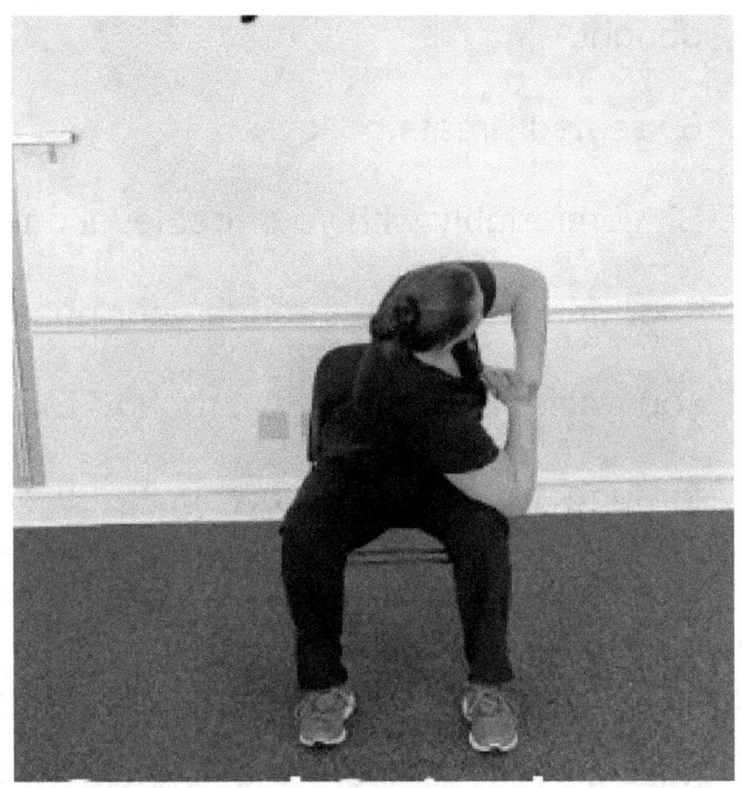

Modification: If twisting is difficult, execute only the arm circles while sitting upright.

6. Seated Breath of Joy:

Sit comfortably with your feet level on the floor. Inhale deeply through your nose as you raise both arms overhead. Exhale through your mouth, producing a "ha" sound, as you lower your arms and lean forward slightly. Inhale again while raising your limbs, and exhale while lowering them.

Modification: If leaning forward is not comfortable, merely raise the arms overhead while breathing deeply.

These exercises can help stimulate blood flow and enhance circulation throughout the body. Remind seniors to breathe deeply and move gently, avoiding any strain. If they have any medical concerns or conditions that affect circulation, encourage them to consult a healthcare professional before attempting new exercises.

Chapter 7

Chair yoga exercises to enhance mind body connections

1. Mindful Breathing:

Sit comfortably in the chair with your spine straight and your hands resting on your lap.Close your eyes and direct your consciousness to your breath. Inhale deeply through your nose, feeling your abdomen rise. Exhale slowly through your lips, feeling your abdomen descend. Focus your attention exclusively on the sensation of your breath as it enters and departs your body.

Modification: Place one hand on the abdomen to feel the rise and fall with each breath, improving awareness of the breath.

2. Seated Body Scan:

Sit comfortably and close your eyes. Slowly devote your attention to different regions of your body, starting with your toes and progressing higher. Notice any sensations, tension, or relaxation in any location without judgment.This technique improves body awareness and relaxation.

Modification: Focus on places that are easier to feel, like the hands, and gradually expand awareness to other parts of the body.

3. Seated Sun Salutations:

Sit comfortably with a straight spine and your hands at your heart. Inhale, raise your arms high, and look up. Exhale and lower your hands back to your heart. WIth each movement, focus on syncing your breath with the motion of your body.

Modification: Use slow and deliberate motions, focusing on the sensation of the stretch as you raise and lower the arms.

4. Seated Heart-Opening Stretch:

Sit at the edge of the chair, placing your hands on your lower back for support. Inhale, softly arch your upper back, and elevate your chest, gazing up slightly. Exhale, release the stretch, and sit upright.Focus on the opening of your chest and heart center.

Modification: If arching is tough, simply focus on stretching the spine and elevating the chest without straining.

5. Seated Mindful Eating:

Choose a little item of food, such as a raisin or a slice of fruit.Bring complete consciousness to the process of eating: observe the texture, flavor, and sensation as you gently chew and swallow.This activity emphasizes mindful eating and presence in the moment.

Modification: If chewing is tough, focus on the scent and texture of the food and savor it slowly.

6. Seated Restorative Pose:

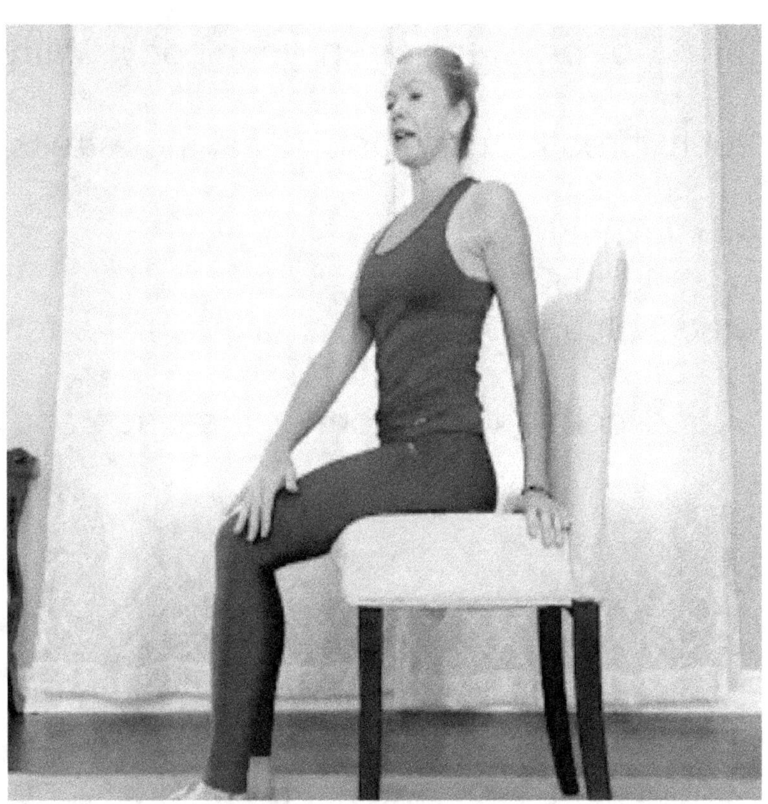

Sit comfortably with your back straight and your feet flat on the floor. Close your eyes and rest your hands on your lap or thighs. Inhale deeply, and as you exhale, let go of any tension in your body. With each breath, consider releasing stress and anxiety.

Modification: Use pillows or cushions for added comfort, supporting the back and neck.

These exercises can help seniors over 60 create a deeper mind-body connection, boosting calm, attention, and self-awareness. Encourage them to approach these practices with an open and non-judgmental attitude. If they find it tough at first, remind them that creating this connection requires time and practice.

Chapter 8

Chair yoga exercises for fitness accessibilities

1. Seated Marching:

Sit at the edge of the chair with your feet flat on the floor.Lift one knee up towards your chest and then lower it down.Alternate legs in a marching motion, activating your core.

Modification: For people with restricted mobility, merely lift the heels off the ground, or alternatively, create a marching motion while keeping the feet on the floor.

2. Seated leg lifts:

Sit comfortably with your feet level on the floor and your hands resting on your thighs.Lift one leg straight out in front of you, holding it for a few breaths.Lower the leg and repeat with the opposite leg.Modification: For people with restricted flexibility, lift the leg as far as is comfortable, even if it's only a few inches above the ground.

3. Seated knee extensions:

Sit with a straight spine and your feet flat on the floor. Extend one leg out in front of you, then flex your foot back.Hold for a moment and release, then switch to the other leg.Modification: Use a resistance band around the foot to make the action simpler, or maintain the knee slightly bent if complete extension is tough.

4. Seated Rowing Motion:

Sit erect with your feet flat on the floor.Hold your hands out in front of you at shoulder height.Pretend you're holding oars and alternate pulling one hand back while extending the other.Modification: For those with limited arm mobility, do the motion with fewer motions and a reduced range of motion.

5. Seated Arm Circles:

Sit comfortably and extend your arms out to the sides. Make tiny circles with your arms in both directions. This exercise helps improve shoulder flexibility and strengthens the arm muscles.

Modification: If shoulder mobility is limited, reduce the size of the circles and focus on the movement that is comfortable.

6. Seated Core Twist:

Sit with a straight spine and your feet flat on the floor. Hold onto the sides of the chair for support. Inhale as you stretch your spine, and as you exhale, gently twist your torso to one side.Inhale to center and exhale to twist to the other side.

Modification: Hold onto the chair's sides for support and complete the twist to a comfortable range.

7. Seated Diaphragmatic Breathing:

Sit comfortably with your spine straight and your hands resting on your lap.Breathe deeply into your diaphragm, allowing your abdomen to rise with each inhalation and sink with each exhalation.This activity improves relaxation and oxygenates the body.

Modification: If this is tough, focus on calm, deep breaths without thinking too much about the rise and fall of the abdomen.

Conclusion

In the realm of chair yoga, the voyage of exploration, self-care, and well-being reaches its glorious end. As we've studied the specialized exercises intended with seniors over 60 in mind, we've entered into a realm of gentle movements, mindfulness, and rejuvenation. Each position, each breath, and each moment of introspection has been a step towards developing flexibility, strengthening the body, and nurturing the spirit.

Chair yoga isn't just about physical poses; it's a symphony of elegance that harmonizes the body, mind, and spirit. The support of the chair becomes a trusted partner, allowing us to embrace the practice with confidence and joy. And as we've woven these activities into our daily routines, we've found a sanctuary of well-being that transcends age, building a connection to our inner energy.

As the practice draws to a close, remember that chair yoga is a journey without an end. It's a route you can travel upon whenever you seek a moment of repair, a breath of peace, or a stretch towards greater flexibility. The lessons of chair yoga transcend beyond the constraints of the chair, reminding us that movement, mindfulness, and self-care are crucial threads in the tapestry of a full and fulfilling life.

So, whether you're starting your journey anew or continuing the route you've accepted, know that chair yoga stands as a beacon of wellbeing, ready to guide you with its gentle wisdom. As you rise from your chair, may you carry the essence of this exercise with you—within every stride, every breath, and every wonderful moment that lies ahead.

Acknowledgments

I would like to convey my heartfelt gratitude to all those who contributed to the preparation of this chair yoga guide for seniors over 60. This undertaking would not have been feasible without the joint efforts, thoughts, and dedication of several individuals.

I am tremendously thankful to the professionals and practitioners who gave their skills and wisdom in the domain of chair yoga. Your guidance has been crucial in structuring the content and ensuring its accuracy.

A special thank you goes to the seniors who participated in testing and developing the chair yoga routines. Your important feedback and experiences have given a depth of authenticity and relevance to this book.

I am appreciative of the healthcare specialists who contributed their views and ideas to ensure that the activities described are safe and effective for people over 60, especially those with unique health considerations.

I would also like to show my appreciation to the creative minds who developed the graphics and illustrations that accompany this book, even if I can't display them here.

Last but not least, a sincere thank you to everyone who contributed support, encouragement, and inspiration during the process. Your belief in the necessity of improving wellness and well-being among seniors has been a driving factor.

To all these individuals and to anyone who has helped in ways known and unseen, I send my heartfelt acknowledgment. This guide stands as a joint effort, a monument to the power of community and shared knowledge.

With gratitude,

Lara Curran